My Personal MS Wellness book

Tracking, Learning and Living

By DeeDee Rupkey

~~~

In This Book:

This book is designed to be a quick reference for you, your doctors and those who care for you – those who love you ☺.

In the very beginning you will find a relapse plan of action. Here you will list your support people, your doctors, your medications and other things that caregivers and/or doctors will need to know.

Next you will find a section filled with boxes for you to fill in about exercise. I could have filled this in for you but let's face it – we are all different – so what works for me may not work for you. There are 12 blank spaces for you to fill in with the exercises that benefit you the most. You can write it is, glue pictures in or whatever else works for you☺

The third and last section is the quick reference wellness checklist for you, your caregivers and your doctors. Let's say you have been using the book for 3 months – now you can really just glance at your book when your doctor asks you how you have been doing! Better yet- you can hand him your book! Seriously- however you choose to do it will work just fine. It tracks the date, exercises, medication, pain, fog/confusion, moods, stress, spasticity and vision in a quick and simple manner. We already have enough on our plates to remember to do right? This makes tracking your major MS symptoms quick and easy! ☺ And it works for a whole year!

It is my sincere hope that this wellness book will help you, your caregivers and your doctors with tracking your wellness.

Light & Love

DeeDee Rupkey

MY RELAPSE PLAN OF ACTION:

(A guide for me and my memory – and those who love me ☺)

Use a Pencil or erasable pen in case of changes

Who are my support people?

Name	Phone Number

My Doctors/Therapists:

Name	Profession	Phone Number

My Medications/Supplements:

Name	Dosage	Frequency	Reason

What generally helps me best in relapse? (help those who love you help you):

_____
_____
_____
_____
_____
_____
_____
_____

Things I may need: (Cane, walker, braces etc… where are they?)

_____
_____
_____
_____
_____
_____
_____

Important things to know: (for those who love me ☺)

_____
_____
_____
_____
_____
_____
_____
_____
_____
_____
_____
_____
_____

EXERCISE REFERENCE

** Add Photos or Instructions of Exercises that work for you**

DAILY WELLNESS TRACKING:

Scale 1-10 – 1 is always great / 10 is always worst

Example

Date:	Exercised? Y/N	Took Meds? Y/N
01/01/2014	**Y**	**Y**
Pain: 1-10	**Fog/Confusion: 1-10**	**Stress: 1-10**
4	**3**	**3**
Mood: 1-10	**Spasticity: 1-10**	**Vision? blurry/good..etc**
3	**4**	**Good**

Date:	Exercised? Y/N	Took Meds? Y/N
Pain: 1-10	Fog/Confusion: 1-10	Stress: 1-10
Mood: 1-10	Spasticity: 1-10	Vision? blurry/good..etc

Date:	Exercised? Y/N	Took Meds? Y/N
Pain: 1-10	Fog/Confusion: 1-10	Stress: 1-10
Mood: 1-10	Spasticity: 1-10	Vision? blurry/good..etc

Date:	Exercised? Y/N	Took Meds? Y/N
Pain: 1-10	Fog/Confusion: 1-10	Stress: 1-10
Mood: 1-10	Spasticity: 1-10	Vision? blurry/good..etc

Date:	Exercised? Y/N	Took Meds? Y/N
Pain: 1-10	Fog/Confusion: 1-10	Stress: 1-10
Mood: 1-10	Spasticity: 1-10	Vision? blurry/good..etc

Date:	Exercised? Y/N	Took Meds? Y/N
Pain: 1-10	Fog/Confusion: 1-10	Stress: 1-10
Mood: 1-10	Spasticity: 1-10	Vision? blurry/good..etc

Date:	Exercised? Y/N	Took Meds? Y/N
Pain: 1-10	Fog/Confusion: 1-10	Stress: 1-10
Mood: 1-10	Spasticity: 1-10	Vision? blurry/good..etc

Date:	Exercised? Y/N	Took Meds? Y/N
Pain: 1-10	Fog/Confusion: 1-10	Stress: 1-10
Mood: 1-10	Spasticity: 1-10	Vision? blurry/good..etc

Date:	Exercised? Y/N	Took Meds? Y/N
Pain: 1-10	Fog/Confusion: 1-10	Stress: 1-10
Mood: 1-10	Spasticity: 1-10	Vision? blurry/good..etc

Date:	Exercised? Y/N	Took Meds? Y/N
Pain: 1-10	Fog/Confusion: 1-10	Stress: 1-10
Mood: 1-10	Spasticity: 1-10	Vision? blurry/good..etc

Date:	Exercised? Y/N	Took Meds? Y/N
Pain: 1-10	Fog/Confusion: 1-10	Stress: 1-10
Mood: 1-10	Spasticity: 1-10	Vision? blurry/good..etc

Date:	Exercised? Y/N	Took Meds? Y/N
Pain: 1-10	Fog/Confusion: 1-10	Stress: 1-10
Mood: 1-10	Spasticity: 1-10	Vision? blurry/good..etc

Date:	Exercised? Y/N	Took Meds? Y/N
Pain: 1-10	Fog/Confusion: 1-10	Stress: 1-10
Mood: 1-10	Spasticity: 1-10	Vision? blurry/good..etc

Date:	Exercised? Y/N	Took Meds? Y/N
Pain: 1-10	Fog/Confusion: 1-10	Stress: 1-10
Mood: 1-10	Spasticity: 1-10	Vision? blurry/good..etc

Date:	Exercised? Y/N	Took Meds? Y/N
Pain: 1-10	Fog/Confusion: 1-10	Stress: 1-10
Mood: 1-10	Spasticity: 1-10	Vision? blurry/good..etc

Date:	Exercised? Y/N	Took Meds? Y/N
Pain: 1-10	Fog/Confusion: 1-10	Stress: 1-10
Mood: 1-10	Spasticity: 1-10	Vision? blurry/good..etc

Date:	Exercised? Y/N	Took Meds? Y/N
Pain: 1-10	Fog/Confusion: 1-10	Stress: 1-10
Mood: 1-10	Spasticity: 1-10	Vision? blurry/good..etc

Date:	Exercised? Y/N	Took Meds? Y/N
Pain: 1-10	Fog/Confusion: 1-10	Stress: 1-10
Mood: 1-10	Spasticity: 1-10	Vision? blurry/good..etc

Date:	Exercised? Y/N	Took Meds? Y/N
Pain: 1-10	Fog/Confusion: 1-10	Stress: 1-10
Mood: 1-10	Spasticity: 1-10	Vision? blurry/good..etc

Date:	Exercised? Y/N	Took Meds? Y/N
Pain: 1-10	Fog/Confusion: 1-10	Stress: 1-10
Mood: 1-10	Spasticity: 1-10	Vision? blurry/good..etc

Date:	Exercised? Y/N	Took Meds? Y/N
Pain: 1-10	Fog/Confusion: 1-10	Stress: 1-10
Mood: 1-10	Spasticity: 1-10	Vision? blurry/good..etc

Date:	Exercised? Y/N	Took Meds? Y/N
Pain: 1-10	Fog/Confusion: 1-10	Stress: 1-10
Mood: 1-10	Spasticity: 1-10	Vision? blurry/good..etc

Date:	Exercised? Y/N	Took Meds? Y/N
Pain: 1-10	Fog/Confusion: 1-10	Stress: 1-10
Mood: 1-10	Spasticity: 1-10	Vision? blurry/good..etc

Date:	Exercised? Y/N	Took Meds? Y/N
Pain: 1-10	Fog/Confusion: 1-10	Stress: 1-10
Mood: 1-10	Spasticity: 1-10	Vision? blurry/good..etc

Date:	Exercised? Y/N	Took Meds? Y/N
Pain: 1-10	Fog/Confusion: 1-10	Stress: 1-10
Mood: 1-10	Spasticity: 1-10	Vision? blurry/good..etc

Date:	Exercised? Y/N	Took Meds? Y/N
Pain: 1-10	Fog/Confusion: 1-10	Stress: 1-10
Mood: 1-10	Spasticity: 1-10	Vision? blurry/good..etc

Date:	Exercised? Y/N	Took Meds? Y/N
Pain: 1-10	Fog/Confusion: 1-10	Stress: 1-10
Mood: 1-10	Spasticity: 1-10	Vision? blurry/good..etc

Date:	Exercised? Y/N	Took Meds? Y/N
Pain: 1-10	Fog/Confusion: 1-10	Stress: 1-10
Mood: 1-10	Spasticity: 1-10	Vision? blurry/good..etc

Date:	Exercised? Y/N	Took Meds? Y/N
Pain: 1-10	Fog/Confusion: 1-10	Stress: 1-10
Mood: 1-10	Spasticity: 1-10	Vision? blurry/good..etc

Date:	Exercised? Y/N	Took Meds? Y/N
Pain: 1-10	Fog/Confusion: 1-10	Stress: 1-10
Mood: 1-10	Spasticity: 1-10	Vision? blurry/good..etc

Date:	Exercised? Y/N	Took Meds? Y/N
Pain: 1-10	Fog/Confusion: 1-10	Stress: 1-10
Mood: 1-10	Spasticity: 1-10	Vision? blurry/good..etc

Date:	Exercised? Y/N	Took Meds? Y/N
Pain: 1-10	Fog/Confusion: 1-10	Stress: 1-10
Mood: 1-10	Spasticity: 1-10	Vision? blurry/good..etc

Date:	Exercised? Y/N	Took Meds? Y/N
Pain: 1-10	Fog/Confusion: 1-10	Stress: 1-10
Mood: 1-10	Spasticity: 1-10	Vision? blurry/good..etc

Date:	Exercised? Y/N	Took Meds? Y/N
Pain: 1-10	Fog/Confusion: 1-10	Stress: 1-10
Mood: 1-10	Spasticity: 1-10	Vision? blurry/good..etc

Date:	Exercised? Y/N	Took Meds? Y/N
Pain: 1-10	Fog/Confusion: 1-10	Stress: 1-10
Mood: 1-10	Spasticity: 1-10	Vision? blurry/good..etc

Date:	Exercised? Y/N	Took Meds? Y/N
Pain: 1-10	Fog/Confusion: 1-10	Stress: 1-10
Mood: 1-10	Spasticity: 1-10	Vision? blurry/good..etc

Date:	Exercised? Y/N	Took Meds? Y/N
Pain: 1-10	Fog/Confusion: 1-10	Stress: 1-10
Mood: 1-10	Spasticity: 1-10	Vision? blurry/good..etc

Date:	Exercised? Y/N	Took Meds? Y/N
Pain: 1-10	Fog/Confusion: 1-10	Stress: 1-10
Mood: 1-10	Spasticity: 1-10	Vision? blurry/good..etc

Date:	Exercised? Y/N	Took Meds? Y/N
Pain: 1-10	Fog/Confusion: 1-10	Stress: 1-10
Mood: 1-10	Spasticity: 1-10	Vision? blurry/good..etc

Date:	Exercised? Y/N	Took Meds? Y/N
Pain: 1-10	Fog/Confusion: 1-10	Stress: 1-10
Mood: 1-10	Spasticity: 1-10	Vision? blurry/good..etc

Date:	Exercised? Y/N	Took Meds? Y/N
Pain: 1-10	Fog/Confusion: 1-10	Stress: 1-10
Mood: 1-10	Spasticity: 1-10	Vision? blurry/good..etc

Date:	Exercised? Y/N	Took Meds? Y/N
Pain: 1-10	Fog/Confusion: 1-10	Stress: 1-10
Mood: 1-10	Spasticity: 1-10	Vision? blurry/good..etc

Date:	Exercised? Y/N	Took Meds? Y/N
Pain: 1-10	Fog/Confusion: 1-10	Stress: 1-10
Mood: 1-10	Spasticity: 1-10	Vision? blurry/good..etc

Date:	Exercised? Y/N	Took Meds? Y/N
Pain: 1-10	Fog/Confusion: 1-10	Stress: 1-10
Mood: 1-10	Spasticity: 1-10	Vision? blurry/good..etc

Date:	Exercised? Y/N	Took Meds? Y/N
Pain: 1-10	Fog/Confusion: 1-10	Stress: 1-10
Mood: 1-10	Spasticity: 1-10	Vision? blurry/good..etc

Date:	Exercised? Y/N	Took Meds? Y/N
Pain: 1-10	Fog/Confusion: 1-10	Stress: 1-10
Mood: 1-10	Spasticity: 1-10	Vision? blurry/good..etc

Date:	Exercised? Y/N	Took Meds? Y/N
Pain: 1-10	Fog/Confusion: 1-10	Stress: 1-10
Mood: 1-10	Spasticity: 1-10	Vision? blurry/good..etc

Date:	Exercised? Y/N	Took Meds? Y/N
Pain: 1-10	Fog/Confusion: 1-10	Stress: 1-10
Mood: 1-10	Spasticity: 1-10	Vision? blurry/good..etc

Date:	Exercised? Y/N	Took Meds? Y/N
Pain: 1-10	Fog/Confusion: 1-10	Stress: 1-10
Mood: 1-10	Spasticity: 1-10	Vision? blurry/good..etc

Date:	Exercised? Y/N	Took Meds? Y/N
Pain: 1-10	Fog/Confusion: 1-10	Stress: 1-10
Mood: 1-10	Spasticity: 1-10	Vision? blurry/good..etc

Date:	Exercised? Y/N	Took Meds? Y/N
Pain: 1-10	Fog/Confusion: 1-10	Stress: 1-10
Mood: 1-10	Spasticity: 1-10	Vision? blurry/good..etc

Date:	Exercised? Y/N	Took Meds? Y/N
Pain: 1-10	Fog/Confusion: 1-10	Stress: 1-10
Mood: 1-10	Spasticity: 1-10	Vision? blurry/good..etc

Date:	Exercised? Y/N	Took Meds? Y/N
Pain: 1-10	Fog/Confusion: 1-10	Stress: 1-10
Mood: 1-10	Spasticity: 1-10	Vision? blurry/good..etc

Date:	Exercised? Y/N	Took Meds? Y/N
Pain: 1-10	Fog/Confusion: 1-10	Stress: 1-10
Mood: 1-10	Spasticity: 1-10	Vision? blurry/good..etc

Date:	Exercised? Y/N	Took Meds? Y/N
Pain: 1-10	Fog/Confusion: 1-10	Stress: 1-10
Mood: 1-10	Spasticity: 1-10	Vision? blurry/good..etc

Date:	Exercised? Y/N	Took Meds? Y/N
Pain: 1-10	Fog/Confusion: 1-10	Stress: 1-10
Mood: 1-10	Spasticity: 1-10	Vision? blurry/good..etc

Date:	Exercised? Y/N	Took Meds? Y/N
Pain: 1-10	Fog/Confusion: 1-10	Stress: 1-10
Mood: 1-10	Spasticity: 1-10	Vision? blurry/good..etc

Date:	Exercised? Y/N	Took Meds? Y/N
Pain: 1-10	Fog/Confusion: 1-10	Stress: 1-10
Mood: 1-10	Spasticity: 1-10	Vision? blurry/good..etc

Date:	Exercised? Y/N	Took Meds? Y/N
Pain: 1-10	Fog/Confusion: 1-10	Stress: 1-10
Mood: 1-10	Spasticity: 1-10	Vision? blurry/good..etc

Date:	Exercised? Y/N	Took Meds? Y/N
Pain: 1-10	Fog/Confusion: 1-10	Stress: 1-10
Mood: 1-10	Spasticity: 1-10	Vision? blurry/good..etc

Date:	Exercised? Y/N	Took Meds? Y/N
Pain: 1-10	Fog/Confusion: 1-10	Stress: 1-10
Mood: 1-10	Spasticity: 1-10	Vision? blurry/good..etc

Date:	Exercised? Y/N	Took Meds? Y/N
Pain: 1-10	Fog/Confusion: 1-10	Stress: 1-10
Mood: 1-10	Spasticity: 1-10	Vision? blurry/good..etc

Date:	Exercised? Y/N	Took Meds? Y/N
Pain: 1-10	Fog/Confusion: 1-10	Stress: 1-10
Mood: 1-10	Spasticity: 1-10	Vision? blurry/good..etc

Date:	Exercised? Y/N	Took Meds? Y/N
Pain: 1-10	Fog/Confusion: 1-10	Stress: 1-10
Mood: 1-10	Spasticity: 1-10	Vision? blurry/good..etc

Date:	Exercised? Y/N	Took Meds? Y/N
Pain: 1-10	Fog/Confusion: 1-10	Stress: 1-10
Mood: 1-10	Spasticity: 1-10	Vision? blurry/good..etc

Date:	Exercised? Y/N	Took Meds? Y/N
Pain: 1-10	Fog/Confusion: 1-10	Stress: 1-10
Mood: 1-10	Spasticity: 1-10	Vision? blurry/good..etc

Date:	Exercised? Y/N	Took Meds? Y/N
Pain: 1-10	Fog/Confusion: 1-10	Stress: 1-10
Mood: 1-10	Spasticity: 1-10	Vision? blurry/good..etc

Date:	Exercised? Y/N	Took Meds? Y/N
Pain: 1-10	Fog/Confusion: 1-10	Stress: 1-10
Mood: 1-10	Spasticity: 1-10	Vision? blurry/good..etc

Date:	Exercised? Y/N	Took Meds? Y/N
Pain: 1-10	Fog/Confusion: 1-10	Stress: 1-10
Mood: 1-10	Spasticity: 1-10	Vision? blurry/good..etc

Date:	Exercised? Y/N	Took Meds? Y/N
Pain: 1-10	Fog/Confusion: 1-10	Stress: 1-10
Mood: 1-10	Spasticity: 1-10	Vision? blurry/good..etc

Date:	Exercised? Y/N	Took Meds? Y/N
Pain: 1-10	Fog/Confusion: 1-10	Stress: 1-10
Mood: 1-10	Spasticity: 1-10	Vision? blurry/good..etc

Date:	Exercised? Y/N	Took Meds? Y/N
Pain: 1-10	Fog/Confusion: 1-10	Stress: 1-10
Mood: 1-10	Spasticity: 1-10	Vision? blurry/good..etc

Date:	Exercised? Y/N	Took Meds? Y/N
Pain: 1-10	Fog/Confusion: 1-10	Stress: 1-10
Mood: 1-10	Spasticity: 1-10	Vision? blurry/good..etc

Date:	Exercised? Y/N	Took Meds? Y/N
Pain: 1-10	Fog/Confusion: 1-10	Stress: 1-10
Mood: 1-10	Spasticity: 1-10	Vision? blurry/good..etc

Date:	Exercised? Y/N	Took Meds? Y/N
Pain: 1-10	Fog/Confusion: 1-10	Stress: 1-10
Mood: 1-10	Spasticity: 1-10	Vision? blurry/good..etc

Date:	Exercised? Y/N	Took Meds? Y/N
Pain: 1-10	Fog/Confusion: 1-10	Stress: 1-10
Mood: 1-10	Spasticity: 1-10	Vision? blurry/good..etc

Date:	Exercised? Y/N	Took Meds? Y/N
Pain: 1-10	Fog/Confusion: 1-10	Stress: 1-10
Mood: 1-10	Spasticity: 1-10	Vision? blurry/good..etc

Date:	Exercised? Y/N	Took Meds? Y/N
Pain: 1-10	Fog/Confusion: 1-10	Stress: 1-10
Mood: 1-10	Spasticity: 1-10	Vision? blurry/good..etc

Date:	Exercised? Y/N	Took Meds? Y/N
Pain: 1-10	Fog/Confusion: 1-10	Stress: 1-10
Mood: 1-10	Spasticity: 1-10	Vision? blurry/good..etc

Date:	Exercised? Y/N	Took Meds? Y/N
Pain: 1-10	Fog/Confusion: 1-10	Stress: 1-10
Mood: 1-10	Spasticity: 1-10	Vision? blurry/good..etc

Date:	Exercised? Y/N	Took Meds? Y/N
Pain: 1-10	Fog/Confusion: 1-10	Stress: 1-10
Mood: 1-10	Spasticity: 1-10	Vision? blurry/good..etc

Date:	Exercised? Y/N	Took Meds? Y/N
Pain: 1-10	Fog/Confusion: 1-10	Stress: 1-10
Mood: 1-10	Spasticity: 1-10	Vision? blurry/good..etc

Date:	Exercised? Y/N	Took Meds? Y/N
Pain: 1-10	Fog/Confusion: 1-10	Stress: 1-10
Mood: 1-10	Spasticity: 1-10	Vision? blurry/good..etc

Date:	Exercised? Y/N	Took Meds? Y/N
Pain: 1-10	Fog/Confusion: 1-10	Stress: 1-10
Mood: 1-10	Spasticity: 1-10	Vision? blurry/good..etc

Date:	Exercised? Y/N	Took Meds? Y/N
Pain: 1-10	Fog/Confusion: 1-10	Stress: 1-10
Mood: 1-10	Spasticity: 1-10	Vision? blurry/good..etc

Date:	Exercised? Y/N	Took Meds? Y/N
Pain: 1-10	Fog/Confusion: 1-10	Stress: 1-10
Mood: 1-10	Spasticity: 1-10	Vision? blurry/good..etc

Date:	Exercised? Y/N	Took Meds? Y/N
Pain: 1-10	Fog/Confusion: 1-10	Stress: 1-10
Mood: 1-10	Spasticity: 1-10	Vision? blurry/good..etc

Date:	Exercised? Y/N	Took Meds? Y/N
Pain: 1-10	Fog/Confusion: 1-10	Stress: 1-10
Mood: 1-10	Spasticity: 1-10	Vision? blurry/good..etc

Date:	Exercised? Y/N	Took Meds? Y/N
Pain: 1-10	Fog/Confusion: 1-10	Stress: 1-10
Mood: 1-10	Spasticity: 1-10	Vision? blurry/good..etc

Date:	Exercised? Y/N	Took Meds? Y/N
Pain: 1-10	Fog/Confusion: 1-10	Stress: 1-10
Mood: 1-10	Spasticity: 1-10	Vision? blurry/good..etc

Date:	Exercised? Y/N	Took Meds? Y/N
Pain: 1-10	Fog/Confusion: 1-10	Stress: 1-10
Mood: 1-10	Spasticity: 1-10	Vision? blurry/good..etc

Date:	Exercised? Y/N	Took Meds? Y/N
Pain: 1-10	Fog/Confusion: 1-10	Stress: 1-10
Mood: 1-10	Spasticity: 1-10	Vision? blurry/good..etc

Date:	Exercised? Y/N	Took Meds? Y/N
Pain: 1-10	Fog/Confusion: 1-10	Stress: 1-10
Mood: 1-10	Spasticity: 1-10	Vision? blurry/good..etc

Date:	Exercised? Y/N	Took Meds? Y/N
Pain: 1-10	Fog/Confusion: 1-10	Stress: 1-10
Mood: 1-10	Spasticity: 1-10	Vision? blurry/good..etc

Date:	Exercised? Y/N	Took Meds? Y/N
Pain: 1-10	Fog/Confusion: 1-10	Stress: 1-10
Mood: 1-10	Spasticity: 1-10	Vision? blurry/good..etc

Date:	Exercised? Y/N	Took Meds? Y/N
Pain: 1-10	Fog/Confusion: 1-10	Stress: 1-10
Mood: 1-10	Spasticity: 1-10	Vision? blurry/good..etc

Date:	Exercised? Y/N	Took Meds? Y/N
Pain: 1-10	Fog/Confusion: 1-10	Stress: 1-10
Mood: 1-10	Spasticity: 1-10	Vision? blurry/good..etc

Date:	Exercised? Y/N	Took Meds? Y/N
Pain: 1-10	Fog/Confusion: 1-10	Stress: 1-10
Mood: 1-10	Spasticity: 1-10	Vision? blurry/good..etc

Date:	Exercised? Y/N	Took Meds? Y/N
Pain: 1-10	Fog/Confusion: 1-10	Stress: 1-10
Mood: 1-10	Spasticity: 1-10	Vision? blurry/good..etc

Date:	Exercised? Y/N	Took Meds? Y/N
Pain: 1-10	Fog/Confusion: 1-10	Stress: 1-10
Mood: 1-10	Spasticity: 1-10	Vision? blurry/good..etc

Date:	Exercised? Y/N	Took Meds? Y/N
Pain: 1-10	Fog/Confusion: 1-10	Stress: 1-10
Mood: 1-10	Spasticity: 1-10	Vision? blurry/good..etc

Date:	Exercised? Y/N	Took Meds? Y/N
Pain: 1-10	Fog/Confusion: 1-10	Stress: 1-10
Mood: 1-10	Spasticity: 1-10	Vision? blurry/good..etc

Date:	Exercised? Y/N	Took Meds? Y/N
Pain: 1-10	Fog/Confusion: 1-10	Stress: 1-10
Mood: 1-10	Spasticity: 1-10	Vision? blurry/good..etc

Date:	Exercised? Y/N	Took Meds? Y/N
Pain: 1-10	Fog/Confusion: 1-10	Stress: 1-10
Mood: 1-10	Spasticity: 1-10	Vision? blurry/good..etc

Date:	Exercised? Y/N	Took Meds? Y/N
Pain: 1-10	Fog/Confusion: 1-10	Stress: 1-10
Mood: 1-10	Spasticity: 1-10	Vision? blurry/good..etc

Date:	Exercised? Y/N	Took Meds? Y/N
Pain: 1-10	Fog/Confusion: 1-10	Stress: 1-10
Mood: 1-10	Spasticity: 1-10	Vision? blurry/good..etc

Date:	Exercised? Y/N	Took Meds? Y/N
Pain: 1-10	Fog/Confusion: 1-10	Stress: 1-10
Mood: 1-10	Spasticity: 1-10	Vision? blurry/good..etc

Date:	Exercised? Y/N	Took Meds? Y/N
Pain: 1-10	Fog/Confusion: 1-10	Stress: 1-10
Mood: 1-10	Spasticity: 1-10	Vision? blurry/good..etc

Date:	Exercised? Y/N	Took Meds? Y/N
Pain: 1-10	Fog/Confusion: 1-10	Stress: 1-10
Mood: 1-10	Spasticity: 1-10	Vision? blurry/good..etc

Date:	Exercised? Y/N	Took Meds? Y/N
Pain: 1-10	Fog/Confusion: 1-10	Stress: 1-10
Mood: 1-10	Spasticity: 1-10	Vision? blurry/good..etc

Date:	Exercised? Y/N	Took Meds? Y/N
Pain: 1-10	Fog/Confusion: 1-10	Stress: 1-10
Mood: 1-10	Spasticity: 1-10	Vision? blurry/good..etc

Date:	Exercised? Y/N	Took Meds? Y/N
Pain: 1-10	Fog/Confusion: 1-10	Stress: 1-10
Mood: 1-10	Spasticity: 1-10	Vision? blurry/good..etc

Date:	Exercised? Y/N	Took Meds? Y/N
Pain: 1-10	Fog/Confusion: 1-10	Stress: 1-10
Mood: 1-10	Spasticity: 1-10	Vision? blurry/good..etc

Date:	Exercised? Y/N	Took Meds? Y/N
Pain: 1-10	Fog/Confusion: 1-10	Stress: 1-10
Mood: 1-10	Spasticity: 1-10	Vision? blurry/good..etc

Date:	Exercised? Y/N	Took Meds? Y/N
Pain: 1-10	Fog/Confusion: 1-10	Stress: 1-10
Mood: 1-10	Spasticity: 1-10	Vision? blurry/good..etc

Date:	Exercised? Y/N	Took Meds? Y/N
Pain: 1-10	Fog/Confusion: 1-10	Stress: 1-10
Mood: 1-10	Spasticity: 1-10	Vision? blurry/good..etc

Date:	Exercised? Y/N	Took Meds? Y/N
Pain: 1-10	Fog/Confusion: 1-10	Stress: 1-10
Mood: 1-10	Spasticity: 1-10	Vision? blurry/good..etc

Date:	Exercised? Y/N	Took Meds? Y/N
Pain: 1-10	Fog/Confusion: 1-10	Stress: 1-10
Mood: 1-10	Spasticity: 1-10	Vision? blurry/good..etc

Date:	Exercised? Y/N	Took Meds? Y/N
Pain: 1-10	Fog/Confusion: 1-10	Stress: 1-10
Mood: 1-10	Spasticity: 1-10	Vision? blurry/good..etc

Date:	Exercised? Y/N	Took Meds? Y/N
Pain: 1-10	Fog/Confusion: 1-10	Stress: 1-10
Mood: 1-10	Spasticity: 1-10	Vision? blurry/good..etc

Date:	Exercised? Y/N	Took Meds? Y/N
Pain: 1-10	Fog/Confusion: 1-10	Stress: 1-10
Mood: 1-10	Spasticity: 1-10	Vision? blurry/good..etc

Date:	Exercised? Y/N	Took Meds? Y/N
Pain: 1-10	Fog/Confusion: 1-10	Stress: 1-10
Mood: 1-10	Spasticity: 1-10	Vision? blurry/good..etc

Date:	Exercised? Y/N	Took Meds? Y/N
Pain: 1-10	Fog/Confusion: 1-10	Stress: 1-10
Mood: 1-10	Spasticity: 1-10	Vision? blurry/good..etc

Date:	Exercised? Y/N	Took Meds? Y/N
Pain: 1-10	Fog/Confusion: 1-10	Stress: 1-10
Mood: 1-10	Spasticity: 1-10	Vision? blurry/good..etc

Date:	Exercised? Y/N	Took Meds? Y/N
Pain: 1-10	Fog/Confusion: 1-10	Stress: 1-10
Mood: 1-10	Spasticity: 1-10	Vision? blurry/good..etc

Date:	Exercised? Y/N	Took Meds? Y/N
Pain: 1-10	Fog/Confusion: 1-10	Stress: 1-10
Mood: 1-10	Spasticity: 1-10	Vision? blurry/good..etc

Date:	Exercised? Y/N	Took Meds? Y/N
Pain: 1-10	Fog/Confusion: 1-10	Stress: 1-10
Mood: 1-10	Spasticity: 1-10	Vision? blurry/good..etc

Date:	Exercised? Y/N	Took Meds? Y/N
Pain: 1-10	Fog/Confusion: 1-10	Stress: 1-10
Mood: 1-10	Spasticity: 1-10	Vision? blurry/good..etc

Date:	Exercised? Y/N	Took Meds? Y/N
Pain: 1-10	Fog/Confusion: 1-10	Stress: 1-10
Mood: 1-10	Spasticity: 1-10	Vision? blurry/good..etc

Date:	Exercised? Y/N	Took Meds? Y/N
Pain: 1-10	Fog/Confusion: 1-10	Stress: 1-10
Mood: 1-10	Spasticity: 1-10	Vision? blurry/good..etc

Date:	Exercised? Y/N	Took Meds? Y/N
Pain: 1-10	Fog/Confusion: 1-10	Stress: 1-10
Mood: 1-10	Spasticity: 1-10	Vision? blurry/good..etc

Date:	Exercised? Y/N	Took Meds? Y/N
Pain: 1-10	Fog/Confusion: 1-10	Stress: 1-10
Mood: 1-10	Spasticity: 1-10	Vision? blurry/good..etc

Date:	Exercised? Y/N	Took Meds? Y/N
Pain: 1-10	Fog/Confusion: 1-10	Stress: 1-10
Mood: 1-10	Spasticity: 1-10	Vision? blurry/good..etc

Date:	Exercised? Y/N	Took Meds? Y/N
Pain: 1-10	Fog/Confusion: 1-10	Stress: 1-10
Mood: 1-10	Spasticity: 1-10	Vision? blurry/good..etc

Date:	Exercised? Y/N	Took Meds? Y/N
Pain: 1-10	Fog/Confusion: 1-10	Stress: 1-10
Mood: 1-10	Spasticity: 1-10	Vision? blurry/good..etc

Date:	Exercised? Y/N	Took Meds? Y/N
Pain: 1-10	Fog/Confusion: 1-10	Stress: 1-10
Mood: 1-10	Spasticity: 1-10	Vision? blurry/good..etc

Date:	Exercised? Y/N	Took Meds? Y/N
Pain: 1-10	Fog/Confusion: 1-10	Stress: 1-10
Mood: 1-10	Spasticity: 1-10	Vision? blurry/good..etc

Date:	Exercised? Y/N	Took Meds? Y/N
Pain: 1-10	Fog/Confusion: 1-10	Stress: 1-10
Mood: 1-10	Spasticity: 1-10	Vision? blurry/good..etc

Date:	Exercised? Y/N	Took Meds? Y/N
Pain: 1-10	Fog/Confusion: 1-10	Stress: 1-10
Mood: 1-10	Spasticity: 1-10	Vision? blurry/good..etc

Date:	Exercised? Y/N	Took Meds? Y/N
Pain: 1-10	Fog/Confusion: 1-10	Stress: 1-10
Mood: 1-10	Spasticity: 1-10	Vision? blurry/good..etc

Date:	Exercised? Y/N	Took Meds? Y/N
Pain: 1-10	Fog/Confusion: 1-10	Stress: 1-10
Mood: 1-10	Spasticity: 1-10	Vision? blurry/good..etc

Date:	Exercised? Y/N	Took Meds? Y/N
Pain: 1-10	Fog/Confusion: 1-10	Stress: 1-10
Mood: 1-10	Spasticity: 1-10	Vision? blurry/good..etc

Date:	Exercised? Y/N	Took Meds? Y/N
Pain: 1-10	Fog/Confusion: 1-10	Stress: 1-10
Mood: 1-10	Spasticity: 1-10	Vision? blurry/good..etc

Date:	Exercised? Y/N	Took Meds? Y/N
Pain: 1-10	Fog/Confusion: 1-10	Stress: 1-10
Mood: 1-10	Spasticity: 1-10	Vision? blurry/good..etc

Date:	Exercised? Y/N	Took Meds? Y/N
Pain: 1-10	Fog/Confusion: 1-10	Stress: 1-10
Mood: 1-10	Spasticity: 1-10	Vision? blurry/good..etc

Date:	Exercised? Y/N	Took Meds? Y/N
Pain: 1-10	Fog/Confusion: 1-10	Stress: 1-10
Mood: 1-10	Spasticity: 1-10	Vision? blurry/good..etc

Date:	Exercised? Y/N	Took Meds? Y/N
Pain: 1-10	Fog/Confusion: 1-10	Stress: 1-10
Mood: 1-10	Spasticity: 1-10	Vision? blurry/good..etc

Date:	Exercised? Y/N	Took Meds? Y/N
Pain: 1-10	Fog/Confusion: 1-10	Stress: 1-10
Mood: 1-10	Spasticity: 1-10	Vision? blurry/good..etc

Date:	Exercised? Y/N	Took Meds? Y/N
Pain: 1-10	Fog/Confusion: 1-10	Stress: 1-10
Mood: 1-10	Spasticity: 1-10	Vision? blurry/good..etc

Date:	Exercised? Y/N	Took Meds? Y/N
Pain: 1-10	Fog/Confusion: 1-10	Stress: 1-10
Mood: 1-10	Spasticity: 1-10	Vision? blurry/good..etc

Date:	Exercised? Y/N	Took Meds? Y/N
Pain: 1-10	Fog/Confusion: 1-10	Stress: 1-10
Mood: 1-10	Spasticity: 1-10	Vision? blurry/good..etc

Date:	Exercised? Y/N	Took Meds? Y/N
Pain: 1-10	Fog/Confusion: 1-10	Stress: 1-10
Mood: 1-10	Spasticity: 1-10	Vision? blurry/good..etc

Date:	Exercised? Y/N	Took Meds? Y/N
Pain: 1-10	Fog/Confusion: 1-10	Stress: 1-10
Mood: 1-10	Spasticity: 1-10	Vision? blurry/good..etc

Date:	Exercised? Y/N	Took Meds? Y/N
Pain: 1-10	Fog/Confusion: 1-10	Stress: 1-10
Mood: 1-10	Spasticity: 1-10	Vision? blurry/good..etc

Date:	Exercised? Y/N	Took Meds? Y/N
Pain: 1-10	Fog/Confusion: 1-10	Stress: 1-10
Mood: 1-10	Spasticity: 1-10	Vision? blurry/good..etc

Date:	Exercised? Y/N	Took Meds? Y/N
Pain: 1-10	Fog/Confusion: 1-10	Stress: 1-10
Mood: 1-10	Spasticity: 1-10	Vision? blurry/good..etc

Date:	Exercised? Y/N	Took Meds? Y/N
Pain: 1-10	Fog/Confusion: 1-10	Stress: 1-10
Mood: 1-10	Spasticity: 1-10	Vision? blurry/good..etc

Date:	Exercised? Y/N	Took Meds? Y/N
Pain: 1-10	Fog/Confusion: 1-10	Stress: 1-10
Mood: 1-10	Spasticity: 1-10	Vision? blurry/good..etc

Date:	Exercised? Y/N	Took Meds? Y/N
Pain: 1-10	Fog/Confusion: 1-10	Stress: 1-10
Mood: 1-10	Spasticity: 1-10	Vision? blurry/good..etc

Date:	Exercised? Y/N	Took Meds? Y/N
Pain: 1-10	Fog/Confusion: 1-10	Stress: 1-10
Mood: 1-10	Spasticity: 1-10	Vision? blurry/good..etc

Date:	Exercised? Y/N	Took Meds? Y/N
Pain: 1-10	Fog/Confusion: 1-10	Stress: 1-10
Mood: 1-10	Spasticity: 1-10	Vision? blurry/good..etc

Date:	Exercised? Y/N	Took Meds? Y/N
Pain: 1-10	Fog/Confusion: 1-10	Stress: 1-10
Mood: 1-10	Spasticity: 1-10	Vision? blurry/good..etc

Date:	Exercised? Y/N	Took Meds? Y/N
Pain: 1-10	Fog/Confusion: 1-10	Stress: 1-10
Mood: 1-10	Spasticity: 1-10	Vision? blurry/good..etc

Date:	Exercised? Y/N	Took Meds? Y/N
Pain: 1-10	Fog/Confusion: 1-10	Stress: 1-10
Mood: 1-10	Spasticity: 1-10	Vision? blurry/good..etc

Date:	Exercised? Y/N	Took Meds? Y/N
Pain: 1-10	Fog/Confusion: 1-10	Stress: 1-10
Mood: 1-10	Spasticity: 1-10	Vision? blurry/good..etc

Date:	Exercised? Y/N	Took Meds? Y/N
Pain: 1-10	Fog/Confusion: 1-10	Stress: 1-10
Mood: 1-10	Spasticity: 1-10	Vision? blurry/good..etc

Date:	Exercised? Y/N	Took Meds? Y/N
Pain: 1-10	Fog/Confusion: 1-10	Stress: 1-10
Mood: 1-10	Spasticity: 1-10	Vision? blurry/good..etc

Date:	Exercised? Y/N	Took Meds? Y/N
Pain: 1-10	Fog/Confusion: 1-10	Stress: 1-10
Mood: 1-10	Spasticity: 1-10	Vision? blurry/good..etc

Date:	Exercised? Y/N	Took Meds? Y/N
Pain: 1-10	Fog/Confusion: 1-10	Stress: 1-10
Mood: 1-10	Spasticity: 1-10	Vision? blurry/good..etc

Date:	Exercised? Y/N	Took Meds? Y/N
Pain: 1-10	Fog/Confusion: 1-10	Stress: 1-10
Mood: 1-10	Spasticity: 1-10	Vision? blurry/good..etc

Date:	Exercised? Y/N	Took Meds? Y/N
Pain: 1-10	Fog/Confusion: 1-10	Stress: 1-10
Mood: 1-10	Spasticity: 1-10	Vision? blurry/good..etc

Date:	Exercised? Y/N	Took Meds? Y/N
Pain: 1-10	Fog/Confusion: 1-10	Stress: 1-10
Mood: 1-10	Spasticity: 1-10	Vision? blurry/good..etc

Date:	Exercised? Y/N	Took Meds? Y/N
Pain: 1-10	Fog/Confusion: 1-10	Stress: 1-10
Mood: 1-10	Spasticity: 1-10	Vision? blurry/good..etc

Date:	Exercised? Y/N	Took Meds? Y/N
Pain: 1-10	Fog/Confusion: 1-10	Stress: 1-10
Mood: 1-10	Spasticity: 1-10	Vision? blurry/good..etc

Date:	Exercised? Y/N	Took Meds? Y/N
Pain: 1-10	Fog/Confusion: 1-10	Stress: 1-10
Mood: 1-10	Spasticity: 1-10	Vision? blurry/good..etc

Date:	Exercised? Y/N	Took Meds? Y/N
Pain: 1-10	Fog/Confusion: 1-10	Stress: 1-10
Mood: 1-10	Spasticity: 1-10	Vision? blurry/good..etc

Date:	Exercised? Y/N	Took Meds? Y/N
Pain: 1-10	Fog/Confusion: 1-10	Stress: 1-10
Mood: 1-10	Spasticity: 1-10	Vision? blurry/good..etc

Date:	Exercised? Y/N	Took Meds? Y/N
Pain: 1-10	Fog/Confusion: 1-10	Stress: 1-10
Mood: 1-10	Spasticity: 1-10	Vision? blurry/good..etc

Date:	Exercised? Y/N	Took Meds? Y/N
Pain: 1-10	Fog/Confusion: 1-10	Stress: 1-10
Mood: 1-10	Spasticity: 1-10	Vision? blurry/good..etc

Date:	Exercised? Y/N	Took Meds? Y/N
Pain: 1-10	Fog/Confusion: 1-10	Stress: 1-10
Mood: 1-10	Spasticity: 1-10	Vision? blurry/good..etc

Date:	Exercised? Y/N	Took Meds? Y/N
Pain: 1-10	Fog/Confusion: 1-10	Stress: 1-10
Mood: 1-10	Spasticity: 1-10	Vision? blurry/good..etc

Date:	Exercised? Y/N	Took Meds? Y/N
Pain: 1-10	Fog/Confusion: 1-10	Stress: 1-10
Mood: 1-10	Spasticity: 1-10	Vision? blurry/good..etc

Date:	Exercised? Y/N	Took Meds? Y/N
Pain: 1-10	Fog/Confusion: 1-10	Stress: 1-10
Mood: 1-10	Spasticity: 1-10	Vision? blurry/good..etc

Date:	Exercised? Y/N	Took Meds? Y/N
Pain: 1-10	Fog/Confusion: 1-10	Stress: 1-10
Mood: 1-10	Spasticity: 1-10	Vision? blurry/good..etc

Date:	Exercised? Y/N	Took Meds? Y/N
Pain: 1-10	Fog/Confusion: 1-10	Stress: 1-10
Mood: 1-10	Spasticity: 1-10	Vision? blurry/good..etc

Date:	Exercised? Y/N	Took Meds? Y/N
Pain: 1-10	Fog/Confusion: 1-10	Stress: 1-10
Mood: 1-10	Spasticity: 1-10	Vision? blurry/good..etc

Date:	Exercised? Y/N	Took Meds? Y/N
Pain: 1-10	Fog/Confusion: 1-10	Stress: 1-10
Mood: 1-10	Spasticity: 1-10	Vision? blurry/good..etc

Date:	Exercised? Y/N	Took Meds? Y/N
Pain: 1-10	Fog/Confusion: 1-10	Stress: 1-10
Mood: 1-10	Spasticity: 1-10	Vision? blurry/good..etc

Date:	Exercised? Y/N	Took Meds? Y/N
Pain: 1-10	Fog/Confusion: 1-10	Stress: 1-10
Mood: 1-10	Spasticity: 1-10	Vision? blurry/good..etc

Date:	Exercised? Y/N	Took Meds? Y/N
Pain: 1-10	Fog/Confusion: 1-10	Stress: 1-10
Mood: 1-10	Spasticity: 1-10	Vision? blurry/good..etc

Date:	Exercised? Y/N	Took Meds? Y/N
Pain: 1-10	Fog/Confusion: 1-10	Stress: 1-10
Mood: 1-10	Spasticity: 1-10	Vision? blurry/good..etc

Date:	Exercised? Y/N	Took Meds? Y/N
Pain: 1-10	Fog/Confusion: 1-10	Stress: 1-10
Mood: 1-10	Spasticity: 1-10	Vision? blurry/good..etc

Date:	Exercised? Y/N	Took Meds? Y/N
Pain: 1-10	Fog/Confusion: 1-10	Stress: 1-10
Mood: 1-10	Spasticity: 1-10	Vision? blurry/good..etc

Date:	Exercised? Y/N	Took Meds? Y/N
Pain: 1-10	Fog/Confusion: 1-10	Stress: 1-10
Mood: 1-10	Spasticity: 1-10	Vision? blurry/good..etc

Date:	Exercised? Y/N	Took Meds? Y/N
Pain: 1-10	Fog/Confusion: 1-10	Stress: 1-10
Mood: 1-10	Spasticity: 1-10	Vision? blurry/good..etc

Date:	Exercised? Y/N	Took Meds? Y/N
Pain: 1-10	Fog/Confusion: 1-10	Stress: 1-10
Mood: 1-10	Spasticity: 1-10	Vision? blurry/good..etc

Date:	Exercised? Y/N	Took Meds? Y/N
Pain: 1-10	Fog/Confusion: 1-10	Stress: 1-10
Mood: 1-10	Spasticity: 1-10	Vision? blurry/good..etc

Date:	Exercised? Y/N	Took Meds? Y/N
Pain: 1-10	Fog/Confusion: 1-10	Stress: 1-10
Mood: 1-10	Spasticity: 1-10	Vision? blurry/good..etc

Date:	Exercised? Y/N	Took Meds? Y/N
Pain: 1-10	Fog/Confusion: 1-10	Stress: 1-10
Mood: 1-10	Spasticity: 1-10	Vision? blurry/good..etc

Date:	Exercised? Y/N	Took Meds? Y/N
Pain: 1-10	Fog/Confusion: 1-10	Stress: 1-10
Mood: 1-10	Spasticity: 1-10	Vision? blurry/good..etc

Date:	Exercised? Y/N	Took Meds? Y/N
Pain: 1-10	Fog/Confusion: 1-10	Stress: 1-10
Mood: 1-10	Spasticity: 1-10	Vision? blurry/good..etc

Date:	Exercised? Y/N	Took Meds? Y/N
Pain: 1-10	Fog/Confusion: 1-10	Stress: 1-10
Mood: 1-10	Spasticity: 1-10	Vision? blurry/good..etc

Date:	Exercised? Y/N	Took Meds? Y/N
Pain: 1-10	Fog/Confusion: 1-10	Stress: 1-10
Mood: 1-10	Spasticity: 1-10	Vision? blurry/good..etc

Date:	Exercised? Y/N	Took Meds? Y/N
Pain: 1-10	Fog/Confusion: 1-10	Stress: 1-10
Mood: 1-10	Spasticity: 1-10	Vision? blurry/good..etc

Date:	Exercised? Y/N	Took Meds? Y/N
Pain: 1-10	Fog/Confusion: 1-10	Stress: 1-10
Mood: 1-10	Spasticity: 1-10	Vision? blurry/good..etc

Date:	Exercised? Y/N	Took Meds? Y/N
Pain: 1-10	Fog/Confusion: 1-10	Stress: 1-10
Mood: 1-10	Spasticity: 1-10	Vision? blurry/good..etc

Date:	Exercised? Y/N	Took Meds? Y/N
Pain: 1-10	Fog/Confusion: 1-10	Stress: 1-10
Mood: 1-10	Spasticity: 1-10	Vision? blurry/good..etc

Date:	Exercised? Y/N	Took Meds? Y/N
Pain: 1-10	Fog/Confusion: 1-10	Stress: 1-10
Mood: 1-10	Spasticity: 1-10	Vision? blurry/good..etc

Date:	Exercised? Y/N	Took Meds? Y/N
Pain: 1-10	Fog/Confusion: 1-10	Stress: 1-10
Mood: 1-10	Spasticity: 1-10	Vision? blurry/good..etc

Date:	Exercised? Y/N	Took Meds? Y/N
Pain: 1-10	Fog/Confusion: 1-10	Stress: 1-10
Mood: 1-10	Spasticity: 1-10	Vision? blurry/good..etc

Date:	Exercised? Y/N	Took Meds? Y/N
Pain: 1-10	Fog/Confusion: 1-10	Stress: 1-10
Mood: 1-10	Spasticity: 1-10	Vision? blurry/good..etc

Date:	Exercised? Y/N	Took Meds? Y/N
Pain: 1-10	Fog/Confusion: 1-10	Stress: 1-10
Mood: 1-10	Spasticity: 1-10	Vision? blurry/good..etc

Date:	Exercised? Y/N	Took Meds? Y/N
Pain: 1-10	Fog/Confusion: 1-10	Stress: 1-10
Mood: 1-10	Spasticity: 1-10	Vision? blurry/good..etc

Date:	Exercised? Y/N	Took Meds? Y/N
Pain: 1-10	Fog/Confusion: 1-10	Stress: 1-10
Mood: 1-10	Spasticity: 1-10	Vision? blurry/good..etc

Date:	Exercised? Y/N	Took Meds? Y/N
Pain: 1-10	Fog/Confusion: 1-10	Stress: 1-10
Mood: 1-10	Spasticity: 1-10	Vision? blurry/good..etc

Date:	Exercised? Y/N	Took Meds? Y/N
Pain: 1-10	Fog/Confusion: 1-10	Stress: 1-10
Mood: 1-10	Spasticity: 1-10	Vision? blurry/good..etc

Date:	Exercised? Y/N	Took Meds? Y/N
Pain: 1-10	Fog/Confusion: 1-10	Stress: 1-10
Mood: 1-10	Spasticity: 1-10	Vision? blurry/good..etc

Date:	Exercised? Y/N	Took Meds? Y/N
Pain: 1-10	Fog/Confusion: 1-10	Stress: 1-10
Mood: 1-10	Spasticity: 1-10	Vision? blurry/good..etc

Date:	Exercised? Y/N	Took Meds? Y/N
Pain: 1-10	Fog/Confusion: 1-10	Stress: 1-10
Mood: 1-10	Spasticity: 1-10	Vision? blurry/good..etc

Date:	Exercised? Y/N	Took Meds? Y/N
Pain: 1-10	Fog/Confusion: 1-10	Stress: 1-10
Mood: 1-10	Spasticity: 1-10	Vision? blurry/good..etc

Date:	Exercised? Y/N	Took Meds? Y/N
Pain: 1-10	Fog/Confusion: 1-10	Stress: 1-10
Mood: 1-10	Spasticity: 1-10	Vision? blurry/good..etc

Date:	Exercised? Y/N	Took Meds? Y/N
Pain: 1-10	Fog/Confusion: 1-10	Stress: 1-10
Mood: 1-10	Spasticity: 1-10	Vision? blurry/good..etc

Date:	Exercised? Y/N	Took Meds? Y/N
Pain: 1-10	Fog/Confusion: 1-10	Stress: 1-10
Mood: 1-10	Spasticity: 1-10	Vision? blurry/good..etc

Date:	Exercised? Y/N	Took Meds? Y/N
Pain: 1-10	Fog/Confusion: 1-10	Stress: 1-10
Mood: 1-10	Spasticity: 1-10	Vision? blurry/good..etc

Date:	Exercised? Y/N	Took Meds? Y/N
Pain: 1-10	Fog/Confusion: 1-10	Stress: 1-10
Mood: 1-10	Spasticity: 1-10	Vision? blurry/good..etc

Date:	Exercised? Y/N	Took Meds? Y/N
Pain: 1-10	Fog/Confusion: 1-10	Stress: 1-10
Mood: 1-10	Spasticity: 1-10	Vision? blurry/good..etc

Date:	Exercised? Y/N	Took Meds? Y/N
Pain: 1-10	Fog/Confusion: 1-10	Stress: 1-10
Mood: 1-10	Spasticity: 1-10	Vision? blurry/good..etc

Date:	Exercised? Y/N	Took Meds? Y/N
Pain: 1-10	Fog/Confusion: 1-10	Stress: 1-10
Mood: 1-10	Spasticity: 1-10	Vision? blurry/good..etc

Date:	Exercised? Y/N	Took Meds? Y/N
Pain: 1-10	Fog/Confusion: 1-10	Stress: 1-10
Mood: 1-10	Spasticity: 1-10	Vision? blurry/good..etc

Date:	Exercised? Y/N	Took Meds? Y/N
Pain: 1-10	Fog/Confusion: 1-10	Stress: 1-10
Mood: 1-10	Spasticity: 1-10	Vision? blurry/good..etc

Date:	Exercised? Y/N	Took Meds? Y/N
Pain: 1-10	Fog/Confusion: 1-10	Stress: 1-10
Mood: 1-10	Spasticity: 1-10	Vision? blurry/good..etc

Date:	Exercised? Y/N	Took Meds? Y/N
Pain: 1-10	Fog/Confusion: 1-10	Stress: 1-10
Mood: 1-10	Spasticity: 1-10	Vision? blurry/good..etc

Date:	Exercised? Y/N	Took Meds? Y/N
Pain: 1-10	Fog/Confusion: 1-10	Stress: 1-10
Mood: 1-10	Spasticity: 1-10	Vision? blurry/good..etc

Date:	Exercised? Y/N	Took Meds? Y/N
Pain: 1-10	Fog/Confusion: 1-10	Stress: 1-10
Mood: 1-10	Spasticity: 1-10	Vision? blurry/good..etc

Date:	Exercised? Y/N	Took Meds? Y/N
Pain: 1-10	Fog/Confusion: 1-10	Stress: 1-10
Mood: 1-10	Spasticity: 1-10	Vision? blurry/good..etc

Date:	Exercised? Y/N	Took Meds? Y/N
Pain: 1-10	Fog/Confusion: 1-10	Stress: 1-10
Mood: 1-10	Spasticity: 1-10	Vision? blurry/good..etc

Date:	Exercised? Y/N	Took Meds? Y/N
Pain: 1-10	Fog/Confusion: 1-10	Stress: 1-10
Mood: 1-10	Spasticity: 1-10	Vision? blurry/good..etc

Date:	Exercised? Y/N	Took Meds? Y/N
Pain: 1-10	Fog/Confusion: 1-10	Stress: 1-10
Mood: 1-10	Spasticity: 1-10	Vision? blurry/good..etc

Date:	Exercised? Y/N	Took Meds? Y/N
Pain: 1-10	Fog/Confusion: 1-10	Stress: 1-10
Mood: 1-10	Spasticity: 1-10	Vision? blurry/good..etc

Date:	Exercised? Y/N	Took Meds? Y/N
Pain: 1-10	Fog/Confusion: 1-10	Stress: 1-10
Mood: 1-10	Spasticity: 1-10	Vision? blurry/good..etc

Date:	Exercised? Y/N	Took Meds? Y/N
Pain: 1-10	Fog/Confusion: 1-10	Stress: 1-10
Mood: 1-10	Spasticity: 1-10	Vision? blurry/good..etc

Date:	Exercised? Y/N	Took Meds? Y/N
Pain: 1-10	Fog/Confusion: 1-10	Stress: 1-10
Mood: 1-10	Spasticity: 1-10	Vision? blurry/good..etc

Date:	Exercised? Y/N	Took Meds? Y/N
Pain: 1-10	Fog/Confusion: 1-10	Stress: 1-10
Mood: 1-10	Spasticity: 1-10	Vision? blurry/good..etc

Date:	Exercised? Y/N	Took Meds? Y/N
Pain: 1-10	Fog/Confusion: 1-10	Stress: 1-10
Mood: 1-10	Spasticity: 1-10	Vision? blurry/good..etc

Date:	Exercised? Y/N	Took Meds? Y/N
Pain: 1-10	Fog/Confusion: 1-10	Stress: 1-10
Mood: 1-10	Spasticity: 1-10	Vision? blurry/good..etc

Date:	Exercised? Y/N	Took Meds? Y/N
Pain: 1-10	Fog/Confusion: 1-10	Stress: 1-10
Mood: 1-10	Spasticity: 1-10	Vision? blurry/good..etc

Date:	Exercised? Y/N	Took Meds? Y/N
Pain: 1-10	Fog/Confusion: 1-10	Stress: 1-10
Mood: 1-10	Spasticity: 1-10	Vision? blurry/good..etc

Date:	Exercised? Y/N	Took Meds? Y/N
Pain: 1-10	Fog/Confusion: 1-10	Stress: 1-10
Mood: 1-10	Spasticity: 1-10	Vision? blurry/good..etc

Date:	Exercised? Y/N	Took Meds? Y/N
Pain: 1-10	Fog/Confusion: 1-10	Stress: 1-10
Mood: 1-10	Spasticity: 1-10	Vision? blurry/good..etc

Date:	Exercised? Y/N	Took Meds? Y/N
Pain: 1-10	Fog/Confusion: 1-10	Stress: 1-10
Mood: 1-10	Spasticity: 1-10	Vision? blurry/good..etc

Date:	Exercised? Y/N	Took Meds? Y/N
Pain: 1-10	Fog/Confusion: 1-10	Stress: 1-10
Mood: 1-10	Spasticity: 1-10	Vision? blurry/good..etc

Date:	Exercised? Y/N	Took Meds? Y/N
Pain: 1-10	Fog/Confusion: 1-10	Stress: 1-10
Mood: 1-10	Spasticity: 1-10	Vision? blurry/good..etc

Date:	Exercised? Y/N	Took Meds? Y/N
Pain: 1-10	Fog/Confusion: 1-10	Stress: 1-10
Mood: 1-10	Spasticity: 1-10	Vision? blurry/good..etc

Date:	Exercised? Y/N	Took Meds? Y/N
Pain: 1-10	Fog/Confusion: 1-10	Stress: 1-10
Mood: 1-10	Spasticity: 1-10	Vision? blurry/good..etc

Date:	Exercised? Y/N	Took Meds? Y/N
Pain: 1-10	Fog/Confusion: 1-10	Stress: 1-10
Mood: 1-10	Spasticity: 1-10	Vision? blurry/good..etc

Date:	Exercised? Y/N	Took Meds? Y/N
Pain: 1-10	Fog/Confusion: 1-10	Stress: 1-10
Mood: 1-10	Spasticity: 1-10	Vision? blurry/good..etc

Date:	Exercised? Y/N	Took Meds? Y/N
Pain: 1-10	Fog/Confusion: 1-10	Stress: 1-10
Mood: 1-10	Spasticity: 1-10	Vision? blurry/good..etc

Date:	Exercised? Y/N	Took Meds? Y/N
Pain: 1-10	Fog/Confusion: 1-10	Stress: 1-10
Mood: 1-10	Spasticity: 1-10	Vision? blurry/good..etc

Date:	Exercised? Y/N	Took Meds? Y/N
Pain: 1-10	Fog/Confusion: 1-10	Stress: 1-10
Mood: 1-10	Spasticity: 1-10	Vision? blurry/good..etc

Date:	Exercised? Y/N	Took Meds? Y/N
Pain: 1-10	Fog/Confusion: 1-10	Stress: 1-10
Mood: 1-10	Spasticity: 1-10	Vision? blurry/good..etc

Date:	Exercised? Y/N	Took Meds? Y/N
Pain: 1-10	Fog/Confusion: 1-10	Stress: 1-10
Mood: 1-10	Spasticity: 1-10	Vision? blurry/good..etc

Date:	Exercised? Y/N	Took Meds? Y/N
Pain: 1-10	Fog/Confusion: 1-10	Stress: 1-10
Mood: 1-10	Spasticity: 1-10	Vision? blurry/good..etc

Date:	Exercised? Y/N	Took Meds? Y/N
Pain: 1-10	Fog/Confusion: 1-10	Stress: 1-10
Mood: 1-10	Spasticity: 1-10	Vision? blurry/good..etc

Date:	Exercised? Y/N	Took Meds? Y/N
Pain: 1-10	Fog/Confusion: 1-10	Stress: 1-10
Mood: 1-10	Spasticity: 1-10	Vision? blurry/good..etc

Date:	Exercised? Y/N	Took Meds? Y/N
Pain: 1-10	Fog/Confusion: 1-10	Stress: 1-10
Mood: 1-10	Spasticity: 1-10	Vision? blurry/good..etc

Date:	Exercised? Y/N	Took Meds? Y/N
Pain: 1-10	Fog/Confusion: 1-10	Stress: 1-10
Mood: 1-10	Spasticity: 1-10	Vision? blurry/good..etc

Date:	Exercised? Y/N	Took Meds? Y/N
Pain: 1-10	Fog/Confusion: 1-10	Stress: 1-10
Mood: 1-10	Spasticity: 1-10	Vision? blurry/good..etc

Date:	Exercised? Y/N	Took Meds? Y/N
Pain: 1-10	Fog/Confusion: 1-10	Stress: 1-10
Mood: 1-10	Spasticity: 1-10	Vision? blurry/good..etc

Date:	Exercised? Y/N	Took Meds? Y/N
Pain: 1-10	Fog/Confusion: 1-10	Stress: 1-10
Mood: 1-10	Spasticity: 1-10	Vision? blurry/good..etc

Date:	Exercised? Y/N	Took Meds? Y/N
Pain: 1-10	Fog/Confusion: 1-10	Stress: 1-10
Mood: 1-10	Spasticity: 1-10	Vision? blurry/good..etc

Date:	Exercised? Y/N	Took Meds? Y/N
Pain: 1-10	Fog/Confusion: 1-10	Stress: 1-10
Mood: 1-10	Spasticity: 1-10	Vision? blurry/good..etc

Date:	Exercised? Y/N	Took Meds? Y/N
Pain: 1-10	Fog/Confusion: 1-10	Stress: 1-10
Mood: 1-10	Spasticity: 1-10	Vision? blurry/good..etc

Date:	Exercised? Y/N	Took Meds? Y/N
Pain: 1-10	Fog/Confusion: 1-10	Stress: 1-10
Mood: 1-10	Spasticity: 1-10	Vision? blurry/good..etc

Date:	Exercised? Y/N	Took Meds? Y/N
Pain: 1-10	Fog/Confusion: 1-10	Stress: 1-10
Mood: 1-10	Spasticity: 1-10	Vision? blurry/good..etc

Date:	Exercised? Y/N	Took Meds? Y/N
Pain: 1-10	Fog/Confusion: 1-10	Stress: 1-10
Mood: 1-10	Spasticity: 1-10	Vision? blurry/good..etc

Date:	Exercised? Y/N	Took Meds? Y/N
Pain: 1-10	Fog/Confusion: 1-10	Stress: 1-10
Mood: 1-10	Spasticity: 1-10	Vision? blurry/good..etc

Date:	Exercised? Y/N	Took Meds? Y/N
Pain: 1-10	Fog/Confusion: 1-10	Stress: 1-10
Mood: 1-10	Spasticity: 1-10	Vision? blurry/good..etc

Date:	Exercised? Y/N	Took Meds? Y/N
Pain: 1-10	Fog/Confusion: 1-10	Stress: 1-10
Mood: 1-10	Spasticity: 1-10	Vision? blurry/good..etc

Date:	Exercised? Y/N	Took Meds? Y/N
Pain: 1-10	Fog/Confusion: 1-10	Stress: 1-10
Mood: 1-10	Spasticity: 1-10	Vision? blurry/good..etc

Date:	Exercised? Y/N	Took Meds? Y/N
Pain: 1-10	Fog/Confusion: 1-10	Stress: 1-10
Mood: 1-10	Spasticity: 1-10	Vision? blurry/good..etc

Date:	Exercised? Y/N	Took Meds? Y/N
Pain: 1-10	Fog/Confusion: 1-10	Stress: 1-10
Mood: 1-10	Spasticity: 1-10	Vision? blurry/good..etc

Date:	Exercised? Y/N	Took Meds? Y/N
Pain: 1-10	Fog/Confusion: 1-10	Stress: 1-10
Mood: 1-10	Spasticity: 1-10	Vision? blurry/good..etc

Date:	Exercised? Y/N	Took Meds? Y/N
Pain: 1-10	Fog/Confusion: 1-10	Stress: 1-10
Mood: 1-10	Spasticity: 1-10	Vision? blurry/good..etc

Date:	Exercised? Y/N	Took Meds? Y/N
Pain: 1-10	Fog/Confusion: 1-10	Stress: 1-10
Mood: 1-10	Spasticity: 1-10	Vision? blurry/good..etc

Date:	Exercised? Y/N	Took Meds? Y/N
Pain: 1-10	Fog/Confusion: 1-10	Stress: 1-10
Mood: 1-10	Spasticity: 1-10	Vision? blurry/good..etc

Date:	Exercised? Y/N	Took Meds? Y/N
Pain: 1-10	Fog/Confusion: 1-10	Stress: 1-10
Mood: 1-10	Spasticity: 1-10	Vision? blurry/good..etc

Date:	Exercised? Y/N	Took Meds? Y/N
Pain: 1-10	Fog/Confusion: 1-10	Stress: 1-10
Mood: 1-10	Spasticity: 1-10	Vision? blurry/good..etc

Date:	Exercised? Y/N	Took Meds? Y/N
Pain: 1-10	Fog/Confusion: 1-10	Stress: 1-10
Mood: 1-10	Spasticity: 1-10	Vision? blurry/good..etc

Date:	Exercised? Y/N	Took Meds? Y/N
Pain: 1-10	Fog/Confusion: 1-10	Stress: 1-10
Mood: 1-10	Spasticity: 1-10	Vision? blurry/good..etc

Date:	Exercised? Y/N	Took Meds? Y/N
Pain: 1-10	Fog/Confusion: 1-10	Stress: 1-10
Mood: 1-10	Spasticity: 1-10	Vision? blurry/good..etc

Date:	Exercised? Y/N	Took Meds? Y/N
Pain: 1-10	Fog/Confusion: 1-10	Stress: 1-10
Mood: 1-10	Spasticity: 1-10	Vision? blurry/good..etc

Date:	Exercised? Y/N	Took Meds? Y/N
Pain: 1-10	Fog/Confusion: 1-10	Stress: 1-10
Mood: 1-10	Spasticity: 1-10	Vision? blurry/good..etc

Date:	Exercised? Y/N	Took Meds? Y/N
Pain: 1-10	Fog/Confusion: 1-10	Stress: 1-10
Mood: 1-10	Spasticity: 1-10	Vision? blurry/good..etc

Date:	Exercised? Y/N	Took Meds? Y/N
Pain: 1-10	Fog/Confusion: 1-10	Stress: 1-10
Mood: 1-10	Spasticity: 1-10	Vision? blurry/good..etc

Date:	Exercised? Y/N	Took Meds? Y/N
Pain: 1-10	Fog/Confusion: 1-10	Stress: 1-10
Mood: 1-10	Spasticity: 1-10	Vision? blurry/good..etc

Date:	Exercised? Y/N	Took Meds? Y/N
Pain: 1-10	Fog/Confusion: 1-10	Stress: 1-10
Mood: 1-10	Spasticity: 1-10	Vision? blurry/good..etc

Date:	Exercised? Y/N	Took Meds? Y/N
Pain: 1-10	Fog/Confusion: 1-10	Stress: 1-10
Mood: 1-10	Spasticity: 1-10	Vision? blurry/good..etc

Date:	Exercised? Y/N	Took Meds? Y/N
Pain: 1-10	Fog/Confusion: 1-10	Stress: 1-10
Mood: 1-10	Spasticity: 1-10	Vision? blurry/good..etc

Date:	Exercised? Y/N	Took Meds? Y/N
Pain: 1-10	Fog/Confusion: 1-10	Stress: 1-10
Mood: 1-10	Spasticity: 1-10	Vision? blurry/good..etc

Date:	Exercised? Y/N	Took Meds? Y/N
Pain: 1-10	Fog/Confusion: 1-10	Stress: 1-10
Mood: 1-10	Spasticity: 1-10	Vision? blurry/good..etc

Date:	Exercised? Y/N	Took Meds? Y/N
Pain: 1-10	Fog/Confusion: 1-10	Stress: 1-10
Mood: 1-10	Spasticity: 1-10	Vision? blurry/good..etc

Date:	Exercised? Y/N	Took Meds? Y/N
Pain: 1-10	Fog/Confusion: 1-10	Stress: 1-10
Mood: 1-10	Spasticity: 1-10	Vision? blurry/good..etc

Date:	Exercised? Y/N	Took Meds? Y/N
Pain: 1-10	Fog/Confusion: 1-10	Stress: 1-10
Mood: 1-10	Spasticity: 1-10	Vision? blurry/good..etc

Date:	Exercised? Y/N	Took Meds? Y/N
Pain: 1-10	Fog/Confusion: 1-10	Stress: 1-10
Mood: 1-10	Spasticity: 1-10	Vision? blurry/good..etc

Date:	Exercised? Y/N	Took Meds? Y/N
Pain: 1-10	Fog/Confusion: 1-10	Stress: 1-10
Mood: 1-10	Spasticity: 1-10	Vision? blurry/good..etc

Date:	Exercised? Y/N	Took Meds? Y/N
Pain: 1-10	Fog/Confusion: 1-10	Stress: 1-10
Mood: 1-10	Spasticity: 1-10	Vision? blurry/good..etc

Date:	Exercised? Y/N	Took Meds? Y/N
Pain: 1-10	Fog/Confusion: 1-10	Stress: 1-10
Mood: 1-10	Spasticity: 1-10	Vision? blurry/good..etc

Date:	Exercised? Y/N	Took Meds? Y/N
Pain: 1-10	Fog/Confusion: 1-10	Stress: 1-10
Mood: 1-10	Spasticity: 1-10	Vision? blurry/good..etc

Date:	Exercised? Y/N	Took Meds? Y/N
Pain: 1-10	Fog/Confusion: 1-10	Stress: 1-10
Mood: 1-10	Spasticity: 1-10	Vision? blurry/good..etc

Date:	Exercised? Y/N	Took Meds? Y/N
Pain: 1-10	Fog/Confusion: 1-10	Stress: 1-10
Mood: 1-10	Spasticity: 1-10	Vision? blurry/good..etc

Date:	Exercised? Y/N	Took Meds? Y/N
Pain: 1-10	Fog/Confusion: 1-10	Stress: 1-10
Mood: 1-10	Spasticity: 1-10	Vision? blurry/good..etc

Date:	Exercised? Y/N	Took Meds? Y/N
Pain: 1-10	Fog/Confusion: 1-10	Stress: 1-10
Mood: 1-10	Spasticity: 1-10	Vision? blurry/good..etc

Date:	Exercised? Y/N	Took Meds? Y/N
Pain: 1-10	Fog/Confusion: 1-10	Stress: 1-10
Mood: 1-10	Spasticity: 1-10	Vision? blurry/good..etc

Date:	Exercised? Y/N	Took Meds? Y/N
Pain: 1-10	Fog/Confusion: 1-10	Stress: 1-10
Mood: 1-10	Spasticity: 1-10	Vision? blurry/good..etc

Date:	Exercised? Y/N	Took Meds? Y/N
Pain: 1-10	Fog/Confusion: 1-10	Stress: 1-10
Mood: 1-10	Spasticity: 1-10	Vision? blurry/good..etc

Date:	Exercised? Y/N	Took Meds? Y/N
Pain: 1-10	Fog/Confusion: 1-10	Stress: 1-10
Mood: 1-10	Spasticity: 1-10	Vision? blurry/good..etc

Date:	Exercised? Y/N	Took Meds? Y/N
Pain: 1-10	Fog/Confusion: 1-10	Stress: 1-10
Mood: 1-10	Spasticity: 1-10	Vision? blurry/good..etc

Date:	Exercised? Y/N	Took Meds? Y/N
Pain: 1-10	Fog/Confusion: 1-10	Stress: 1-10
Mood: 1-10	Spasticity: 1-10	Vision? blurry/good..etc

Date:	Exercised? Y/N	Took Meds? Y/N
Pain: 1-10	Fog/Confusion: 1-10	Stress: 1-10
Mood: 1-10	Spasticity: 1-10	Vision? blurry/good..etc

Date:	Exercised? Y/N	Took Meds? Y/N
Pain: 1-10	Fog/Confusion: 1-10	Stress: 1-10
Mood: 1-10	Spasticity: 1-10	Vision? blurry/good..etc

Date:	Exercised? Y/N	Took Meds? Y/N
Pain: 1-10	Fog/Confusion: 1-10	Stress: 1-10
Mood: 1-10	Spasticity: 1-10	Vision? blurry/good..etc

Date:	Exercised? Y/N	Took Meds? Y/N
Pain: 1-10	Fog/Confusion: 1-10	Stress: 1-10
Mood: 1-10	Spasticity: 1-10	Vision? blurry/good..etc

Date:	Exercised? Y/N	Took Meds? Y/N
Pain: 1-10	Fog/Confusion: 1-10	Stress: 1-10
Mood: 1-10	Spasticity: 1-10	Vision? blurry/good..etc

Date:	Exercised? Y/N	Took Meds? Y/N
Pain: 1-10	Fog/Confusion: 1-10	Stress: 1-10
Mood: 1-10	Spasticity: 1-10	Vision? blurry/good..etc

Date:	Exercised? Y/N	Took Meds? Y/N
Pain: 1-10	Fog/Confusion: 1-10	Stress: 1-10
Mood: 1-10	Spasticity: 1-10	Vision? blurry/good..etc

Date:	Exercised? Y/N	Took Meds? Y/N
Pain: 1-10	Fog/Confusion: 1-10	Stress: 1-10
Mood: 1-10	Spasticity: 1-10	Vision? blurry/good..etc

Date:	Exercised? Y/N	Took Meds? Y/N
Pain: 1-10	Fog/Confusion: 1-10	Stress: 1-10
Mood: 1-10	Spasticity: 1-10	Vision? blurry/good..etc

Date:	Exercised? Y/N	Took Meds? Y/N
Pain: 1-10	Fog/Confusion: 1-10	Stress: 1-10
Mood: 1-10	Spasticity: 1-10	Vision? blurry/good..etc

Date:	Exercised? Y/N	Took Meds? Y/N
Pain: 1-10	Fog/Confusion: 1-10	Stress: 1-10
Mood: 1-10	Spasticity: 1-10	Vision? blurry/good..etc

Date:	Exercised? Y/N	Took Meds? Y/N
Pain: 1-10	Fog/Confusion: 1-10	Stress: 1-10
Mood: 1-10	Spasticity: 1-10	Vision? blurry/good..etc

Date:	Exercised? Y/N	Took Meds? Y/N
Pain: 1-10	Fog/Confusion: 1-10	Stress: 1-10
Mood: 1-10	Spasticity: 1-10	Vision? blurry/good..etc

Date:	Exercised? Y/N	Took Meds? Y/N
Pain: 1-10	Fog/Confusion: 1-10	Stress: 1-10
Mood: 1-10	Spasticity: 1-10	Vision? blurry/good..etc

Date:	Exercised? Y/N	Took Meds? Y/N
Pain: 1-10	Fog/Confusion: 1-10	Stress: 1-10
Mood: 1-10	Spasticity: 1-10	Vision? blurry/good..etc

Date:	Exercised? Y/N	Took Meds? Y/N
Pain: 1-10	Fog/Confusion: 1-10	Stress: 1-10
Mood: 1-10	Spasticity: 1-10	Vision? blurry/good..etc

Date:	Exercised? Y/N	Took Meds? Y/N
Pain: 1-10	Fog/Confusion: 1-10	Stress: 1-10
Mood: 1-10	Spasticity: 1-10	Vision? blurry/good..etc

Date:	Exercised? Y/N	Took Meds? Y/N
Pain: 1-10	Fog/Confusion: 1-10	Stress: 1-10
Mood: 1-10	Spasticity: 1-10	Vision? blurry/good..etc

Date:	Exercised? Y/N	Took Meds? Y/N
Pain: 1-10	Fog/Confusion: 1-10	Stress: 1-10
Mood: 1-10	Spasticity: 1-10	Vision? blurry/good..etc

Date:	Exercised? Y/N	Took Meds? Y/N
Pain: 1-10	Fog/Confusion: 1-10	Stress: 1-10
Mood: 1-10	Spasticity: 1-10	Vision? blurry/good..etc

Date:	Exercised? Y/N	Took Meds? Y/N
Pain: 1-10	Fog/Confusion: 1-10	Stress: 1-10
Mood: 1-10	Spasticity: 1-10	Vision? blurry/good..etc

Date:	Exercised? Y/N	Took Meds? Y/N
Pain: 1-10	Fog/Confusion: 1-10	Stress: 1-10
Mood: 1-10	Spasticity: 1-10	Vision? blurry/good..etc

Date:	Exercised? Y/N	Took Meds? Y/N
Pain: 1-10	Fog/Confusion: 1-10	Stress: 1-10
Mood: 1-10	Spasticity: 1-10	Vision? blurry/good..etc

Date:	Exercised? Y/N	Took Meds? Y/N
Pain: 1-10	Fog/Confusion: 1-10	Stress: 1-10
Mood: 1-10	Spasticity: 1-10	Vision? blurry/good..etc

Date:	Exercised? Y/N	Took Meds? Y/N
Pain: 1-10	Fog/Confusion: 1-10	Stress: 1-10
Mood: 1-10	Spasticity: 1-10	Vision? blurry/good..etc

Date:	Exercised? Y/N	Took Meds? Y/N
Pain: 1-10	Fog/Confusion: 1-10	Stress: 1-10
Mood: 1-10	Spasticity: 1-10	Vision? blurry/good..etc

Date:	Exercised? Y/N	Took Meds? Y/N
Pain: 1-10	Fog/Confusion: 1-10	Stress: 1-10
Mood: 1-10	Spasticity: 1-10	Vision? blurry/good..etc

Date:	Exercised? Y/N	Took Meds? Y/N
Pain: 1-10	Fog/Confusion: 1-10	Stress: 1-10
Mood: 1-10	Spasticity: 1-10	Vision? blurry/good..etc

Date:	Exercised? Y/N	Took Meds? Y/N
Pain: 1-10	Fog/Confusion: 1-10	Stress: 1-10
Mood: 1-10	Spasticity: 1-10	Vision? blurry/good..etc

Date:	Exercised? Y/N	Took Meds? Y/N
Pain: 1-10	Fog/Confusion: 1-10	Stress: 1-10
Mood: 1-10	Spasticity: 1-10	Vision? blurry/good..etc

Date:	Exercised? Y/N	Took Meds? Y/N
Pain: 1-10	Fog/Confusion: 1-10	Stress: 1-10
Mood: 1-10	Spasticity: 1-10	Vision? blurry/good..etc

Date:	Exercised? Y/N	Took Meds? Y/N
Pain: 1-10	Fog/Confusion: 1-10	Stress: 1-10
Mood: 1-10	Spasticity: 1-10	Vision? blurry/good..etc

Date:	Exercised? Y/N	Took Meds? Y/N
Pain: 1-10	Fog/Confusion: 1-10	Stress: 1-10
Mood: 1-10	Spasticity: 1-10	Vision? blurry/good..etc

Date:	Exercised? Y/N	Took Meds? Y/N
Pain: 1-10	Fog/Confusion: 1-10	Stress: 1-10
Mood: 1-10	Spasticity: 1-10	Vision? blurry/good..etc

Date:	Exercised? Y/N	Took Meds? Y/N
Pain: 1-10	Fog/Confusion: 1-10	Stress: 1-10
Mood: 1-10	Spasticity: 1-10	Vision? blurry/good..etc

Date:	Exercised? Y/N	Took Meds? Y/N
Pain: 1-10	Fog/Confusion: 1-10	Stress: 1-10
Mood: 1-10	Spasticity: 1-10	Vision? blurry/good..etc

Date:	Exercised? Y/N	Took Meds? Y/N
Pain: 1-10	Fog/Confusion: 1-10	Stress: 1-10
Mood: 1-10	Spasticity: 1-10	Vision? blurry/good..etc

Date:	Exercised? Y/N	Took Meds? Y/N
Pain: 1-10	Fog/Confusion: 1-10	Stress: 1-10
Mood: 1-10	Spasticity: 1-10	Vision? blurry/good..etc

Date:	Exercised? Y/N	Took Meds? Y/N
Pain: 1-10	Fog/Confusion: 1-10	Stress: 1-10
Mood: 1-10	Spasticity: 1-10	Vision? blurry/good..etc

Date:	Exercised? Y/N	Took Meds? Y/N
Pain: 1-10	Fog/Confusion: 1-10	Stress: 1-10
Mood: 1-10	Spasticity: 1-10	Vision? blurry/good..etc

Date:	Exercised? Y/N	Took Meds? Y/N
Pain: 1-10	Fog/Confusion: 1-10	Stress: 1-10
Mood: 1-10	Spasticity: 1-10	Vision? blurry/good..etc

Date:	Exercised? Y/N	Took Meds? Y/N
Pain: 1-10	Fog/Confusion: 1-10	Stress: 1-10
Mood: 1-10	Spasticity: 1-10	Vision? blurry/good..etc

Date:	Exercised? Y/N	Took Meds? Y/N
Pain: 1-10	Fog/Confusion: 1-10	Stress: 1-10
Mood: 1-10	Spasticity: 1-10	Vision? blurry/good..etc

Date:	Exercised? Y/N	Took Meds? Y/N
Pain: 1-10	Fog/Confusion: 1-10	Stress: 1-10
Mood: 1-10	Spasticity: 1-10	Vision? blurry/good..etc

Date:	Exercised? Y/N	Took Meds? Y/N
Pain: 1-10	Fog/Confusion: 1-10	Stress: 1-10
Mood: 1-10	Spasticity: 1-10	Vision? blurry/good..etc

Date:	Exercised? Y/N	Took Meds? Y/N
Pain: 1-10	Fog/Confusion: 1-10	Stress: 1-10
Mood: 1-10	Spasticity: 1-10	Vision? blurry/good..etc

☺ I hope this book has helped you ☺